A WOMAN'S GUIDE TO GOOD HEALTH

Empower Your Well-being:"A Woman's Comprehensive Guide to Achieving and Sustaining Good Health"

DR LAUREL SMITH

TABLE OF CONTENTS

INTRODUCTION

CHAPTER ONE
- Understanding the Unique Health Needs of Women
- The Importance of Prioritizing Women's Health

CHAPTER TWO
- Nutrition for Women
- Managing Weight and Body Image

CHAPTER THREE

- Physical Fitness and Exercise
- Building a Sustainable Exercise Routine

CHAPTER FOUR

- Mental Health and Stress Management
- Strategies for Managing Stress and Anxiety

CHAPTER FIVE

- Reproductive Health
- Understanding the Menstrual Cycle
- Contraception Options

- Hormonal Health

CHAPTER SIX

- Healthy Aging
- Promoting Longevity and Vitality
- Anti-aging Strategies
- Coping with Age-Related Changes

CHAPTER SEVEN

- Self-Care and Well-being
- Stress Reduction Techniques
- Building a Supportive Health Network

CHAPTER EIGHT

- Empowering Your Health Choices
- CONCLUSION

INTRODUCTION

In a world where women's roles and responsibilities are continually expanding, it has never been more crucial for women to prioritize their health and well-being. "Empower Your Well-being: A Woman's Comprehensive Guide to Achieving and Sustaining Good Health" is an invitation to embark on a transformative journey towards optimal physical, mental, and emotional health.

As women navigate the diverse challenges of modern life, from career aspirations to family obligations, it's all too easy to overlook one's own health. Yet, the vitality and strength of women are the very foundations upon which families, communities, and societies are built. This guide is designed to empower women with the knowledge and tools necessary to take charge of their health, fostering resilience, balance, and longevity.

Throughout the pages of this guide, we will delve into a wealth of information tailored specifically to the unique needs and experiences of women. From nutrition and fitness to mental health and self-care strategies, we will explore a holistic approach to well-being that encompasses every facet of a woman's life. We will debunk myths, provide evidence-based advice, and offer practical tips to help you make informed choices about your health.

CHAPTER ONE

<u>Understanding the Unique Health Needs of Women</u>

Ladies' wellbeing alludes to the part of medication that spotlights on the treatment and finding of sicknesses and conditions that influence a lady's physical and profound prosperity.

At the point when individuals consider ladies' wellbeing, the principal subjects that frequently struck a chord might be gynecological worries like fruitlessness, menopause, pregnancy and labor. However, these issues are only a portion of the larger picture regarding women's health.
There are numerous challenges and barriers to well-being that women and children face. These reach from the conditions that shape wellbeing including one's business, training, neighborhood and family circumstance to psychological well-being and mortality. "It is essential that we comprehend the obstacles they face because healthy women and children are the foundation of healthy, strong communities everywhere." For the family to stay solid, the lady in that family should be sound. She frequently maintains everyone else's progress toward their health journey and health goals.

"Data show that women have a distinct set of health care concerns and are more likely than men to develop certain diseases and conditions." The health and well-being of women and families across the nation is greatly impacted by these issues.

Late information show patterns in the use of the medical care framework and sickness commonness in view old enough, orientation and identity. A few key discoveries:

Women's bodies undergo significant transformations throughout their lives, resulting in distinct health concerns for various age groups.

Contrasts exist in the use examples and soundness of ladies across identities.

Numerous ladies deal with their own continuous medical issue, yet they likewise assume a significant part in medical services dynamic inside their families and are in many cases answerable for the majority of providing care for kids and maturing relatives.

"Ladies are more uncertain than men to get proceeded with care once they have an ongoing condition conditions like diabetes, coronary illness, persistent lung infection. According to the National Institutes of Health, women in the United States make approximately 80% of the decisions regarding their families' health care. Once men receive that wake-up call, they are more likely to seek treatment for their chronic condition.
"Employers are progressively looking for advantages to assist ladies and their families with things like care navigation, parental journey support and backup childcare,"

<u>Taking up maternal health equity</u>

Globally, the rates of pregnancy-related mortality have decreased as a result of medical progress. Nonetheless, among the wealthy countries of the globe, the United States has one of the highest rates of maternal deaths. Furthermore, Black women are at considerably greater danger.
Black women are three to four times as likely than white or Hispanic mothers to die during delivery. Additionally, a Black mother with a

college degree has a 60% higher chance of dying as a mother than a white or Hispanic woman with only a high school degree. "Employers should be aware that many of the women in your ranks may be undergoing pregnancy; these women may not be experiencing rainbows and butterflies, but rather a genuine fear that they may pass away during theirpregnancy, at the time of delivery, or in the aftermath. A person's capacity to perform their work may be impacted by the weight of that concern.

Employers must foster a psychologically secure environment since it can increase engagement and retention.
"The journey of a human being is incredibly complex." And I believe that one of the things we discovered during the epidemic is that there aren't many lines between your personal and professional lives. Therefore, we must become extremely astute in ensuring that we are prepared to meet each employee's unique demands.

Numerous specializations and areas of interest are included in women's health, including:

gynecology, birth control, and sexually transmitted diseases (STIs)

Ovarian cancer, breast cancer, and other malignancies that affect women

Breast imaging

Menopause in addition tohormone replacement treatment

The osteoporosis

Getting pregnant and giving birth

Sexual well-being

Heart disease in women

benign diseases that impact how well the female reproductive organs operate

<u>The Importance of Prioritizing Women's Health</u>

It's more crucial than ever to put your physical and emotional wellness first. Many women have neglected their basic health and wellbeing needs over the previous several years. Their everyday habits, including how they interact with friends and family, have changed. For some women, the combination has resulted in severe health issues.

It is important for women and girls to consider their unique health requirements and take action to enhance their general health. Now is a perfect time for all women and girls to focus on improved health, whether you maintain your present hobbies or find new ones. This is especially true for individuals with underlying health concerns, such as diabetes, hypertension, obesity, cardiovascular and respiratory disorders, and women 65 years of age and beyond.

Plan your yearly checkups for physicals and other medical appointments
Discuss the following issues with your physician assistant, nurse practitioner, doctor, or nurse;

- The vaccination against COVID-19 as well as any others you might not have received during the outbreak.

- Preventive treatment includes things like PAP smears, mammograms, bone density scans, stress testing, blood pressure checks, physical examinations, cholesterol screenings, and other screenings for preventive health issues that you might have overlooked during the epidemic.

- If managing your everyday tasks is becoming difficult due to stress, anxiety, or sadness.

- If, more than two weeks following the birth of your child, you are experiencing depression, overwhelm, or difficulty sleeping or eating. Postpartum depression might be what you're dealing with.

CHAPTER TWO

Nutrition for Women

You are a lady who is full of energy and a doer! In the hustle and bustle of work and personal obligations, healthy eating habits are frequently neglected. When the body and mind begin to falter, it is finally apparent that there is a nutritional deficit.

Both increasing awareness of this issue and providing women with proper nourishment are crucial. A 1500–2000 calorie daily diet is necessary for a busy woman, as it increases energy and reduces stress. A long-term health maintenance and increased fertility are benefits of a nutrient-rich diet.

Women's nutritional needs are distinct from men's and differ in several aspects. Women can only function at their peak at work or when doing household tasks if they are eating a healthy diet.

For women to live completely and keep their health, a variety of essential nutrients are required. Women's dietary demands are different, as we have already discussed. This contains certain minerals and vitamins that are vital to the health of women. Of these, iron is more important for women than for men since it helps to preserve hemoglobin and reduce blood loss during menstruation. For healthy bones, women also need to consume adequate amounts of calcium and vitamin D. It is crucial to realize that a woman's dietary requirements vary at different stages of her life, including pregnancy, puberty, menopause, and work-related stress. Women may choose their food and nutrition with knowledge if they take these nutritional requirements into account.

The following essential nutrients must be incorporated into the lifestyle of a working woman:

Vitamin Folic Acid

Vitamin B, folic acid, aids in the body's production of new, healthy cells. Vitamin Folic Acid is necessary for women who are expectant. It supports neural tube development in the fetus. Folic acid supplementation helps avoid birth abnormalities.
You may find folic acid in:

greens with leaves

legumes

Cereals for Breakfast

citrus-based cuisine

Brussels sprouts

Vitamin-D

Fat-soluble vitamin D aids in the gut's absorption of calcium and keeps the concentration of calcium and phosphorus in the right amounts for bone mineral density. In addition to being beneficial for bone health, vitamin D can fend off autoimmune disorders and cancer. When sunrays hit the skin, they can start the production of vitamin D.

Vitamin D is present in -

fatty fish, such as tuna, swordfish, and salmon

yolks of eggs

dairy goods

Red meat

Mushroom

Omega Three

Polyunsaturated lipids, or good fats, such omega-3 fatty acids lower the risk of heart disease and promote heart health. Omega-3 fatty acids must be consumed in order to sustain good health because the body is unable to manufacture enough of them. Pregnant and lactating women may also benefit from omega-3 fatty acids.
Sources of omega-3 fatty acids include:

Fatty Fish, such as Sardines and Salmon

Flax Seeds

Chia seeds

COD hepatic fluid

Veggies

Probiotics

Probiotics are a blend of yeast and beneficial bacteria that reside in your body and maintain your health. Microorganisms found in probiotics are meant to aid with digestion and replenish gut flora. They have shown promise in treating lactose intolerance, urinary tract infections, gastrointestinal issues, and vaginal infections.
Probiotics are present in:

Yogurt

Curd

Kefir

Miso

Picks

sourdough bread

Calcium

Calcium is an essential element for healthy teeth and bones. The majority of the calcium in the body gives bones and teeth their structure and hardness. Women are more prone than men to suffer osteoporosis, a disorder that causes the bones to deteriorate. As a result, it's critical that women take calcium supplements to keep their bones healthy and dense.
Foods high in calcium include:

dairy goods

greens with leaves

Almonds

enhanced liquids

Cheese

Any product using fortified flour

Iron

An crucial component of hemoglobin is iron. Red blood cells, which carry oxygen from the lungs to the body's cells, are formed mostly of iron. Iron also supports the health of connective tissues and muscle metabolism. In addition, iron is necessary for the production of hormones, brain development, cellular activity, and physical growth.
Because women lose more blood during their periods, they are more likely to develop iron deficiency anemia. For a healthier life and a stronger physique, it becomes essential for working women and women in general to maintain appropriate iron levels.
Foods high in iron include red meat:

Fish

legumes

Greens with dark leaves

strengthened cereals

Legumes

Nuts and dried fruit

To stay strong and healthy throughout your life, it's critical to provide your body with the proper nutrients, including vitamins and minerals. Iron, calcium, and vitamin D deficiencies can be brought on by unhealthful eating habits.
But fear not—taking care of oneself doesn't have to be a difficult undertaking. You may make sure that your body is healthy by eating meals high in nutrients and taking the recommended supplements.
Since we only have one body, it should be given the respect and care it needs. Recall to prioritize taking care of yourself.

10 Nutritious Food Suggestions for Women

Healthy eating is crucial for a woman's general health and wellbeing. Avoid skipping meals in favor of resisting the impulse to eat unhealthy snacks. As employed women in a tight pace, it might be difficult to find the time to make nutritious meals and snacks. To help you make healthy eating more doable, consider the following diet advice:

1. Make a plan in advance

Make a meal plan for the day in advance. Every day, set aside some time to arrange your necessary diet. Pay attention to your snacks and diet. Meal planning will assist you in staying on course and avoiding bad decisions.

2. When dining out, choose a healthy choice

When dining out, search the menu for selections that are healthful. Toss in some veggies, grilled chicken, salad, and other healthful alternatives for your supper. If you have anything on your menu that you could later regret, balance it out with something nutritious. When placing an order, adjust and make changes if the food products don't meet your demands for a healthy diet.

3. Bring wholesome snacks to work.

Your energy may be depleted to near nothing during labor hours. It's critical to continuously refuel your body with nibbles and little meals. By bringing wholesome snacks to work, you may prevent the chaos that comes with eating poorly and stay motivated throughout the day.
Fruits, almonds, and protein bars are a few healthier power snacks that are worth adding to your box. Fruits, vegetable sticks, and certain entire foods are all possible to carry. Not

only will these little morsels keep you full, but they'll also lift your spirits and help you avoid becoming stressed out at work.

4. Reduce your sugar intake

Sugar can contribute to overeating and weight gain.Diabetes and heart issues are also brought on by sugar. Additionally, sugar is bad for the skin. Sugar isn't really beneficial for anything but taste.

Take only as much sugar as is essential to enhance your flavor and raise your glucose-derived energy levels. If you have a sweet tooth, switch to sweeteners and eat more fruits and vegetables, which are abundant in glucose and have sweet tastes as well. Drink water whenever you want anything sweet.

5. Cook more frequently at home

It might be difficult to schedule time for home cooking. Either ordering takeout or online could appear handy. It's not as nutritious as cooked meals, despite its convenience. A working woman can cook at home to save money, gain control over their nutrition, and eat considerably better. Moreover, you can discover a new pastime if you cook more at home.

6. Consume a range of fruits and vegetables.

Vegetables and fruits have distinct tastes. They are satisfying, flavorful, and healthful. A diet high in vegetables is very beneficial to the health. Fruits are delicious and just as healthful.

The proverb "An apple a day keeps the doctor away" is still applicable today. Vegetables and fruits are excellent snacks that may be had at any time. They are abundant in nutrients. A diet high in fruits and vegetables improves digestion, lowers blood pressure, lowers cholesterol, lowers the risk of heart disease, provides the body with essential nutrients, and prevents cancer.

7. Increase your seafood intake

Choosing nutritious meals when you have a hectic schedule might be difficult. You will, however, commend one healthy decision: adding fish to your meals. Fish is a great way to promote a healthy diet. They are rich in omega-3 fatty acids and a fantastic source of protein.

Take a moment to prepare a fish-based lunch to fuel your body. Try often adding fish to the dish, along with your preferred tastes, and reap the rewards.

8. Eat a diet high in protein and fiber.

Most individuals don't get enough fiber and protein in their diets. An active day requires stamina and strength. Foods strong in fiber and protein are excellent sources of nutrients to keep you active all day.

Foods high in protein, such meat, dairy, eggs, yogurt, and fish, aid in cellular activity, quick muscle recovery, and maintaining body weight. Naturally, foods strong in fiber and low in carbohydrates, such broccoli, almonds, oats, and chia seeds, are beneficial for blood sugar, cholesterol, and intestinal health as well as helping one reach a healthy weight. Including foods high in fiber and protein will keep you alert, limber, and tip-toeing throughout the day.

9. Eat frequently

When you can eat to nourish yourself, why would you choose to miss meals?
Everyone experiences unhealthy, weary, and distracted feelings when they miss meals. Make eating regularly a priority, and you'll see significant gains in your overall health.

Use Vantage Fit to track your meals.

Vantage Circle's employee health app, Vantage Fit, puts people first. It is intended for businesses and women that value fitness, nutrition, and overall well-being, such as yourself. Vantage Fit encourages better habits and lifestyle choices for exercise and preventative health.
Monitoring your diet might be difficult. To make it possible, Vantage Fit offers a catalog with over 4,000 food choices. Important nutritional information is provided by the catalog, including the amount of fat, protein, and carbohydrates in each food item.
Additional features include customizable badges and trophies, a calorie counter, and a BMI calculator. Gift cards and fitness points are two ways that Vantage Fit provides incentives.

With each step, you can learn from and accomplish your objectives with the support of an expanding community focused on fitness and wellbeing.
Make Use Of Vantage Fit and track your meals, monitor your intake, and take charge of your nutrition!

Women's Meal Planning

Planning meals is a great way for staff members to maintain a healthy diet. To make meal planning easier, think about meal preparation and batch cooking. These are some suggestions for making wholesome breakfasts, lunches, and dinners.

Breakfast

The first meal of the day is breakfast. A nutritious meal maintains bodily energy and establishes the tone for the remainder of the day. For a working woman, a nutritious breakfast may consist of the following:

Scrambled Eggs

oats

Egg-filled Chia Seeds

Brown Bread with Condiments

Nuts and Fruits

Complete Grain

Omelet and spinach

Yogurt

Idl

Poha

 Curd Rice

Porridge

Oatmeal with fruits overnight

Tea

Lunch.

Midday retreat, or lunch, is when we take a break from the daily grind. Now is the time to enjoy our favorite dishes. After lunch, we rejuvenate both our bodies and minds for the remainder of the day. For ladies who have hectic schedules, some nutritious lunch alternatives are:

Grilled chicken

Caramelized Veggies

Tuna or Salmon

Avocado on a salad

bread made with whole grains

Dal and rice

Lentils and Chappatis

Green Leafy Vegetables

Grains of brown rice

Quinoa

Pasta made with whole grains

fresh fruit and yogurt

roasted veggie and rice bowl

Rice and Tofu

Paneer served with veggies and roti

Curry with vegetables and chapattis

Supper

Dinner is the last meal of the day and is usually consumed in the evening or at night. People gather together for dinner to enjoy food, stories, and conversation. Dinner is the last meal we have before retiring for the night to rest, replenish our energy reserves, and get some much-needed sleep. Among the nutritious supper choices are:

Sweet Potato and Baked Salmon

Asparagus

Stir-fry tofu

Vibrant Vegetables

Noodles with Zucchini

Soup with lentils

Sweet potatoes baked with black beans

Quinoa and Fish Together

Dal and a rice dish

salad with grilled chicken

soup and vegetable stew

Vegetable stew with rice bowl

Grilled fish and rice

It can be challenging for a working woman to balance her personal and professional lives as well as her nutrition and health objectives. Taking care of everything in life might be difficult. Your dietary requirements, however, must come first if you want to be as healthy and happy as possible. Understanding the specific dietary demands, making good choices, and including meal planning and tracking go a long way in achieving any kind of goal, whether it be professional or personal. Making nutritious food choices is really essential. minor adjustments make significant changes, and putting your diet and health first, along with adopting good habits, will benefit your body and health in many ways—both now and in the road.

Sustain a Healthy Weight

Retaining a healthy weight helps reduce the chance of high blood pressure, diabetes, heart disease, and stroke. It can also reduce the chance of developing a variety of malignancies.

Although everyone has a different definition of a healthy weight, it's crucial to understand what that means for you.

Discuss your health objectives with your physician or nurse, and together, develop a personalized strategy.

Get Moving and Stay Active: One of the most crucial things you can do to enhance your health at any age is to engage in physical activity. Generally speaking, physical exercise is any movement that improves health. This implies that household chores and gardening can be considered forms of physical exertion.

Plan out your weekly activities based on the objective: 150 minutes a week of moderate-intensity aerobic exercise will raise your heart rate.

4. Divide your exercise into manageable chunks. Take a 15- or 30-minute stroll when you have a break. Regular exercise strengthens your heart, and exposure to sunshine's Vitamin D will strengthen your immune system.

5. Incorporating muscle-strengthening exercises, such as weightlifting or resistance band use, can help ward off sarcopenia, or the loss of muscle with age and immobility.

6. Determine a regimen that works for you depending on your age, life stage, and skill level. There are safe methods to exercise while pregnant, but it's crucial to see your doctor before beginning or altering any physical activity.

7. Take Care of Yourself Internally
Consume meals and snacks that are balanced.

8. Eating heart-healthy entails restricting some foods, including added sugars and trans and saturated fats, and favoring others, like fruits and vegetables.

9. Look for ways to guarantee balanced, weight-healthy meals when dining out and at home.

9. It's critical to make sure your food has adequate vitamins.

10. Your body need vitamin D in order to create and maintain strong bones. Calcium absorption occurs exclusively in the presence of vitamin D in the body. The immune system, muscular function, and brain cell activity are all supported by the anti-inflammatory, antioxidant, and neuroprotective qualities of vitamin D. Milk, yogurt,

orange juice, cereals, and oily fish including salmon, rainbow trout, tinned tuna, and sardines are examples of foods that are all excellent providers of vitamin D.

11. Calcium is also essential, particularly for long-term bone health. Dairy products, such as milk, yogurt, cheese, and drinks fortified with calcium like soy and almond milk, are the finest sources of calcium. Dark green leafy vegetables, dried beans and peas, fish with bones, and juices and cereals fortified with calcium are additional sources of calcium.

12. Take Care of Your Mental Health by Self-Caring

13. Write down a list of quick self-care tasks you can complete each day.

14. Check in to determine whether you require assistance or support in going about your everyday life.

15. Maintain contact with loved ones and friends.

16. Establish a connection with neighborhood or religious groups.

17. Set aside time to relax and engage in your favorite hobbies.

18. Assist those who look after others in your life. Give yourself some time if you are a caregiver.

19. Keep an eye out for shifts in your mood

20. Seek assistance if you or anyone you know is going through changes in behavior, mood, or thought patterns that include self-harm:

21. Look for healthy methods for stress relief

22. Prepare a toolkit of natural stress-reduction techniques.

23. Even little, daily activities like setting aside time for reading, yoga, and meditation can help lower stress levels.

24. You can feel more grounded by taking a few minutes to relax in nature, going for a walk, or listening to your favorite music.

<u>Establish healthy sleeping routines</u>

Roughly 50 to 70 million Americans suffer from a sleep issue, and roughly one in three individuals do not consistently obtain the required amount of sleep needed to maintain good health.

Lack of sleep may result in accidents, decreased productivity, increased risk of mortality, and mental and physical health issues like depression and heart disease.

To enhance your sleeping patterns, especially on the weekends, stick to a schedule for going to bed and waking up at the same times every day.

Make an effort to sleep for at least 7 hours.

Keep a sleep journal if you suspect you may have a sleep issue. Sharing the diary with your medical professional can help him or her diagnose a potential sleep problem.

"You can also check out Dr Ruby Russell's book "Overcoming Insomnia" on the Amazon kindle platform ."

What is meant by body image?

An individual's emotional attitudes, beliefs, and impressions about their own body are referred to as their body image. According to experts, it's a complicated emotional experience.Relationships between body image and what someone thinks of their looks their thoughts on their shape, size, weight, and height their perception and interaction with their body.

Negative body image is associated with discontent and the desire for one's body to be different, whereas positive body image is associated with acceptance and contentment with one's body.

Eating disorders, body dysmorphic disorder (BDD), and other diseases can be exacerbated by having a poor body image.

A positive body image: what is it?

A person who has a positive body image is at ease with their physical appearance and has a positive relationship with it.

Positivity about one's physique comprises:

1) Embracing and being grateful for one's physique

2) Possessing a wide definition of beauty

3) Making efforts to take care of one's body

CHAPTER THREE

Physical Fitness and Exercise

Exercise and Physical Fitness for Women Physical fitness is important for women because it lowers the risk of chronic diseases including diabetes, osteoporosis, and heart disease, maintains a healthy weight, and supports cardiovascular health. Additionally, it increases vitality, lowers stress, and enhances mental health.

Exercise Types: To maintain joint health, a well-rounded regimen should incorporate cardiovascular activities (such as walking), flexibility exercises (such as yoga or stretching), and balancing exercises (such as Pilates) to lower the chance of falls and accidents.

Benefits Particular to Women: Exercise can be particularly helpful in regulating hormone levels, reducing PMS and menopausal symptoms, and promoting reproductive health. Additionally, it aids in the fight against despair and anxiety, which are more common among women.When organizing their workout regimens, women should take their age, lifestyle, and any particular health issues into account. It is advisable to speak with a healthcare professional before beginning a new fitness regimen, particularly if you are pregnant or dealing with medical issues.

Building a Sustainable Exercise Routine

Creating a Long-Term Fitness Program for Women Start Slowly: To prevent fatigue and lower the chance of injury, start with modest, manageable goals and progressively increase the length and intensity of exercises.

Consistency Over Intensity: An fitness regimen that can be sustained over time is considered sustainable. Aim for at least 150 minutes of moderate-intensity exercise each week by choosing things you love and incorporating them into your routine.

Balance and Variety: To address all facets of fitness, use a variety of cardio, strength, flexibility, and balance activities. Variety helps keep things interesting.Different muscle groups may be worked and boredom avoided with variety.

Rest and Recovery: Plan days off to give muscles time to heal and avoid overtraining, which can result in weariness and injury.

 Pay Attention to Your Body: Observe any indications of pain or strain, particularly in the vicinity of the joints, and modify the regimen as necessary. If you are uncertain about proper form or technique, seek expert advice.

Realistic Goal-Setting: Whether for weight loss, mental wellness, or health enhancement, establish personal fitness objectives that are clear, quantifiable, and attainable. Progress tracking may be inspiring as well.

 Emphasis on Nutrition: A healthy diet promotes exercise and recuperation. To keep hydrated and invigorated, give priority to complex carbohydrates, proteins, healthy fats, and lots of water.

CHAPTER FOUR

Mental Health and Stress Management

Mental health is essential for overall well-being, but many women face unique challenges due to biological, societal, and life role factors. Women may experience stress related to career pressures, family responsibilities, caregiving roles, and sometimes gender-based expectations, all of which can affect mental health. Common mental health issues for women include anxiety, depression, and stress-related conditions, often heightened during hormonal transitions such as pregnancy, menopause, and menstruation.

Stress management is vital to help women maintain a balanced lifestyle and reduce the negative impact of stress on both mental and physical health. Learning to manage stress can improve mood, relationships, and productivity while reducing risks for health problems like hypertension, heart disease, and insomnia.

Strategies for Managing Stress and Anxiety

1) Mindfulness and Meditation: Practicing mindfulness, meditation, and breathing exercises can help women stay present, reduce anxiety, and cultivate calmness.

2) Physical Activity: Regular exercise releases endorphins, which boost mood and reduce stress. Activities like yoga, walking, or swimming can be particularly beneficial.

3) Social Support: Connecting with friends, family, or support groups provides emotional support and helps reduce feelings of isolation.

4) Time Management: Setting priorities and boundaries to manage time effectively can help women balance personal and professional commitments, reducing overwhelm.

5) Self-Care: Prioritizing self-care, whether through hobbies, rest, or relaxation practices, can enhance resilience and overall well-being.

6) Professional Help: Consulting a therapist, counselor, or mental health professional can provide women with personalized strategies and support to manage stress and anxiety effectively.

7) Healthy Lifestyle Choices: A balanced diet, adequate sleep, and limiting caffeine and alcohol intake can have positive effects on stress levels and mental health.

These strategies can help women proactively manage stress and maintain good mental health, fostering a healthier and more balanced life.

CHAPTER FIVE

Reproductive Health

Reproductive health is a critical aspect of women's overall well-being, encompassing physical, mental, and social factors related to the reproductive system. It includes everything from menstruation and fertility to pregnancy, childbirth, and menopause. Good reproductive health also involves access to healthcare, information on sexual health, safe pregnancy practices, and prevention of diseases or conditions affecting reproductive organs. Proper reproductive health care helps women make informed decisions, maintain a healthy reproductive system, and improve quality of life.

Understanding the Menstrual Cycle

The menstrual cycle is a monthly process that prepares the body for a potential pregnancy. It typically lasts 28 days but can vary from woman to woman. The cycle is divided into four phases: menstruation, the follicular phase, ovulation, and the luteal phase. Hormones like estrogen and progesterone play a significant role in regulating the cycle. Understanding the menstrual cycle can help women track fertility, identify irregularities, and detect health issues. Awareness of this cycle allows women to better manage symptoms like PMS (premenstrual syndrome) and make informed reproductive health choices.

Contraception Options

Contraception allows women to control if and when they become pregnant, providing family planning and reproductive autonomy. There are various contraception options, including:

Hormonal Methods: Birth control pills, patches, injections, and hormonal IUDs regulate hormones to prevent ovulation.

Barrier Methods: Condoms, diaphragms, and cervical caps physically prevent sperm from reaching the egg.

Intrauterine Devices (IUDs): Non-hormonal (copper) IUDs are placed in the uterus to prevent fertilization.

Permanent Methods: Sterilization (like tubal ligation) is a permanent option for women who don't plan to conceive in the future.

Each option has benefits and potential side effects, and choice depends on individual health, lifestyle, and personal preferences.

Hormonal Health

Hormonal health is essential for regulating various body functions, from metabolism and mood to reproductive health. For women, hormonal changes significantly affect menstruation, fertility, pregnancy, and menopause. Imbalances in hormones like estrogen, progesterone, and testosterone can cause issues such as irregular periods, PCOS (polycystic ovary syndrome), mood swings, and low energy. Maintaining hormonal health through balanced nutrition, exercise, sleep, and managing stress can help women avoid many hormone-related health problems. Regular check-ups with healthcare providers can also detect and address hormonal imbalances early.

ChatGPT

You said:
Write short notes on Mental Health and Stress Management For Women And

Strategies for Managing Stress and Anxiety For Women
ChatGPT said:
ChatGPT
Mental Health and Stress Management for Women
Mental health is essential for overall well-being, but many women face unique challenges due to biological, societal, and life role factors. Women may experience stress related to career pressures, family responsibilities, caregiving roles, and sometimes gender-based expectations, all of which can affect mental health. Common mental health issues for women include anxiety, depression, and stress-related conditions, often heightened during hormonal transitions such as pregnancy, menopause, and menstruation.

Stress management is vital to help women maintain a balanced lifestyle and reduce the negative impact of stress on both mental and physical health. Learning to manage stress can improve mood, relationships, and productivity while reducing risks for health problems like hypertension, heart disease, and insomnia.

Strategies for Managing Stress and Anxiety for Women
Mindfulness and Meditation: Practicing mindfulness, meditation, and breathing exercises can help women stay present, reduce anxiety, and cultivate calmness.

Physical Activity: Regular exercise releases endorphins, which boost mood and reduce stress. Activities like yoga, walking, or swimming can be particularly beneficial.

Social Support: Connecting with friends, family, or support groups provides emotional support and helps reduce feelings of isolation.

Time Management: Setting priorities and boundaries to manage time effectively can help women balance personal and professional commitments, reducing overwhelm.

Self-Care: Prioritizing self-care, whether through hobbies, rest, or relaxation practices, can enhance resilience and overall well-being.

Professional Help: Consulting a therapist, counselor, or mental health professional can provide women with personalized strategies and support to manage stress and anxiety effectively.

Healthy Lifestyle Choices: A balanced diet, adequate sleep, and limiting caffeine and alcohol intake can have positive effects on stress levels and mental health.

These strategies can help women proactively manage stress and maintain good mental health, fostering a healthier and more balanced life.

You said:
Write short notes on
Reproductive Health
Understanding the Menstrual Cycle
Contraception Options

Hormonal Health

For women
ChatGPT said:
ChatGPT
Reproductive Health
Reproductive health is a critical aspect of women's overall well-being, encompassing physical, mental, and social factors related to the reproductive system. It includes everything from menstruation and fertility to pregnancy, childbirth, and menopause. Good reproductive health also involves access to healthcare, information on sexual health, safe pregnancy practices, and prevention of diseases or conditions affecting reproductive organs. Proper reproductive health care helps women make informed decisions, maintain a healthy reproductive system, and improve quality of life.

Understanding the Menstrual Cycle
The menstrual cycle is a monthly process that prepares the body for a potential pregnancy. It typically lasts 28 days but can vary from woman to woman. The cycle is divided into four phases: menstruation, the follicular phase, ovulation, and the luteal phase. Hormones like estrogen and progesterone play a significant role in regulating the cycle. Understanding the menstrual cycle can help women track fertility, identify irregularities, and detect health issues. Awareness of this cycle allows women to better manage symptoms like PMS (premenstrual syndrome) and make informed reproductive health choices.

Contraception Options
Contraception allows women to control if and when they become pregnant, providing family planning and reproductive autonomy. There are various contraception options, including:

Hormonal Methods: Birth control pills, patches, injections, and hormonal IUDs regulate hormones to prevent ovulation.
Barrier Methods: Condoms, diaphragms, and cervical caps physically prevent sperm from reaching the egg.

Intrauterine Devices (IUDs): Non-hormonal (copper) IUDs are placed in the uterus to prevent fertilization.

Permanent Methods: Sterilization (like tubal ligation) is a permanent option for women who don't plan to conceive in the future.

Each option has benefits and potential side effects, and choice depends on individual health, lifestyle, and personal preferences.

Hormonal Health

Hormonal health is essential for regulating various body functions, from metabolism and mood to reproductive health. For women, hormonal changes significantly affect menstruation, fertility, pregnancy, and menopause. Imbalances in hormones like estrogen, progesterone, and testosterone can cause issues such as irregular periods, PCOS (polycystic ovary syndrome), mood swings, and low energy. Maintaining hormonal health through balanced nutrition, exercise, sleep, and managing stress can help women avoid many hormone-related health problems. Regular check-ups with healthcare providers can also detect and address hormonal imbalances early.

CHAPTER SIX

Healthy Aging

Healthy aging involves maintaining physical, mental, and emotional well-being as women grow older. As women age, their bodies undergo various changes, such as decreased bone density, slower metabolism, and changes in skin elasticity. Healthy aging emphasizes habits that support longevity, such as regular exercise, a balanced diet, mental stimulation, and preventive healthcare. Women who adopt these habits early on are more likely to age with vitality and independence, while reducing risks of age-related diseases.

Promoting Longevity and Vitality

Longevity and vitality are achievable through consistent lifestyle practices that promote overall health. For women, this can include eating a nutrient-rich diet, prioritizing cardiovascular health, staying socially connected, and engaging in activities that stimulate the mind. Additionally, regular health screenings, especially for conditions like osteoporosis, heart disease, and cancer, are essential to catch and manage potential health risks early. Physical activity, mental engagement, and social support also play vital roles in sustaining energy levels and preserving quality of life.

Anti-aging Strategies

Anti-aging strategies focus on preserving health and appearance as women age. This can include skincare routines to protect against sun damage, hydration, and using antioxidants. Beyond skincare, anti-aging strategies often emphasize balanced hormone levels, which can be achieved through lifestyle or medical options, and a diet rich in anti-inflammatory foods. Exercise and strength training are also effective for keeping bones strong and reducing muscle loss, which becomes more prevalent with age. Overall, these strategies help women age gracefully, feeling and looking their best.

Coping with Age-Related Changes

Aging brings various changes, including shifts in physical abilities, hormone levels, and sometimes, mental processing speed. Coping with these changes requires both acceptance and proactive management. This may include learning new ways to manage stress, staying socially active to prevent isolation, and adapting physical routines to accommodate new limits or risks. Support from family, friends, or counselors can provide emotional strength, while routine health screenings can help women anticipate and address changes effectively. Coping strategies allow women to embrace aging while continuing to live fulfilling and active lives.

CHAPTER SEVEN

Self-Care and Well-being

Self-care is essential for maintaining well-being, especially for women who often juggle multiple roles in family, career, and community. Self-care involves intentionally taking time to care for mental, emotional, and physical health. Activities can range from setting aside time for relaxation and hobbies to maintaining a healthy diet, regular exercise, and getting enough sleep. Practicing self-care enables women to recharge, reduce stress, and build resilience, ultimately enhancing overall well-being and quality of life.

Stress Reduction Techniques

Effective stress reduction techniques can help women manage the pressures of daily life. Popular methods include mindfulness meditation, deep breathing exercises, and physical activity like yoga or walking, which release tension and improve mood. Journaling, setting boundaries, and time management are also valuable ways to reduce stress. Prioritizing stress reduction helps women maintain emotional balance, boost mental clarity, and prevent long-term health issues linked to chronic stress, such as heart disease and anxiety.

Building a Supportive Health Network

A supportive health network gives women access to the resources, guidance, and encouragement they need to maintain good health. This network can include healthcare providers, family, friends, and support groups. Women benefit from having a primary care physician, mental health professional, and possibly specialists for reproductive or hormonal health. Building a strong support network ensures that women can seek advice, receive preventive care, and feel supported in managing health challenges. A positive health network also provides emotional support and can significantly improve mental well-being.

CHAPTER EIGHT

Empowering Your Health Choices for Women

Empowering health choices is about women taking active control over their physical, mental, and emotional well-being. It involves understanding personal health needs, making informed decisions, and setting health goals that align with one's lifestyle and values. Empowerment in health begins with education—learning about conditions that affect women uniquely, such as reproductive health, hormonal balance, and age-related changes. Knowledge about preventive care, nutrition, exercise, and mental wellness allows women to make choices that support long-term vitality.

Empowering health choices also means advocating for oneself within healthcare settings. Women are encouraged to seek healthcare providers who listen to their concerns, discuss options openly, and respect their preferences. Asking questions, seeking second opinions when necessary, and understanding treatment options are key steps. When women are well-informed, they are more confident in managing conditions, following treatment plans, and prioritizing their health.

Building a health-supportive lifestyle is also part of empowerment, encompassing balanced nutrition, regular physical activity, mental health care, and stress management. By taking these actions, women can feel more in control of their health outcomes and resilient against life's challenges. Health empowerment encourages women to honor their well-being as a lifelong priority, enhancing quality of life and overall self-fulfillment.

CONCLUSION

In conclusion, "A Woman's Guide To Good Health" seeks to empower, inform, and inspire women to take control of their well-being across every stage of life. From understanding reproductive health and managing stress to navigating age-related changes, this guide emphasizes that health is not just the absence of illness it's a holistic state of physical, mental, and emotional balance. Each chapter underscores the importance of proactive choices, self-awareness, and a supportive network as pillars for sustaining health and vitality.

As you embark on your journey toward optimal well-being, remember that caring for your health is an investment in every aspect of your life. It's about honoring your body, nurturing your mind, and cultivating resilience to meet life's challenges with strength and grace. Empowered with knowledge, you are equipped to make decisions that align with your needs, values, and dreams.

Let this guide serve as a foundation for building a life of health, confidence, and joy a life where you prioritize yourself, embrace your uniqueness, and thrive.

9 7 9 8 3 4 6 0 3 2 5 8 8